PESCATARIAN COOKBOOK

Guide On Eating A Well Balanced
Meal For A Healthy Lifestyle

Stephanie J. Watts

Table of Contents

INTRODUCTION

A type of diet known as pescatarianism emphasizes eating fish and seafood in addition to fruits, vegetables, grains, and legumes. It is a popular option for those who want to eat fish and seafood but avoid meat from other animals like cows, pigs, and chickens. Pescatarians may likewise follow a plant-based diet yet at the same time consume creature consume dairy items and eggs, making it protein. Pescatarians commonly stay away from meat like hamburger, chicken, and pork, as well as creature items like eggs and dairy.

CHAPTER1

The significances of pescatarian diet

The fact that pescatarianism is distinct from a vegetarian or vegan diet is one of its primary advantages. Due to the health benefits of eating fish and the growing awareness of its potential to improve heart health, this dietary lifestyle is gaining popularity. Seafood and fish are about sustainability and animal welfare.

The high levels of omega-3 fatty acids found in fish are one of the main advantages of an omega-3-

rich vegetarian diet. Omega-3 fatty acids are necessary for preventing and maintaining heart health. It has been demonstrated that some types lower the risk of heart disease and stroke. Additionally, pescatarians typically eat a diet low in fish, including salmon, mackerel, and tuna. Tuna, which is especially rich in omega-3 fatty acids, is an essential part of a pescatarian's diet. Additionally, fish is a low-fat protein source.

Pescatarianism's potential to improve the environment is yet another advantage. Modern domesticated animals cultivating is a significant supporter of ozone depleting substance outflows and deforestation, though fish and fish can be more maintainable choices. By deciding to eat fish rather than meat, pescatarians can assist with decreasing their carbon impression and backing more is many times lower in soaked fat than other creature proteins.

While embracing a pescatarian diet, guaranteeing that the fish and feasible food fish systems is significant.

Being a consumOverallled are, sustainablyesc sourcedatar.ian Overism is a diet that is adaptable, healthy, and free of destructive fishing methods for people who want to eat animal protein but still put sustainability and plant-based foods first. A decline in fish populations has occurred as a result of the wide variety of fish and seafood available, and choosing to eat fish that is sourced sustainably can support responsible fishing practices. Pescatarians should be aware that not all seafood is created equal when it comes to enjoying a varied and flavorful diet without jeopardizing their own health or the health of the planet. sustainability, with some species facing greater threats of extinction than others. A pescatarian diet can ensure that it is beneficial not only for one's own health but also for the health of the planet by educating oneself on sustainable seafood practices.

In general, pescatarianism is a way of eating that encourages sustainable and responsible food consumption and has the potential to provide numerous health benefits. Pescatarians can support responsible fishing practices and maintain a healthy heart by consuming fish and seafood as their primary source of protein. When deciding to follow a pescatarian diet, it's important to think about sustainability and where food comes from. However, if you have the right information, it can be an enjoyable and rewarding lifestyle.

CHAPTER2

Pescatarianism is a dietary way of life that includes the utilization of fish and fish as the essential wellspring of creature protein. The pescatarian diet is frequently followed for environmental sustainability, ethical issues, or health concerns. This diet is like a veggie lover or vegetarian way of life, however with the expansion of fish. Pescatarians avoid eating all types of meat, including beef, pork, lamb, and poultry.

The pescatarian diet comprises of different fish and fish, including salmon, fish, shrimp, lobster, and crab. Plant-based foods like nuts, seeds, fruits, and vegetables are also eaten by pescatarians. This diet is wealthy in omega-3 unsaturated fats, which are fundamental for keeping up with heart wellbeing, lessening aggravation, and further developing cerebrum capability. Pescatarians also eat a lot of protein, vitamins, and minerals, so their diet is healthy and balanced.

The pescatarian diet is both environmentally friendly and long-lasting. Seafood and fish typically come from sustainable fisheries, which has less of an effect on marine ecosystems. Additionally, pescatarianism encourages the consumption of plant-based foods, thereby decreasing the demand for products derived from animals, which have a significant negative impact on the environment. A pescatarian diet can support ethical and sustainable food practices while also providing numerous health benefits.

Pescatarianism is a way of eating that includes seafood, fish, and foods made from plants. Pescatarians don't eat poultry or meat. The standards of pescatarianism depend on the conviction that a plant-based diet, in blend with fish and fish, is a solid and supportable approach to everyday life. This way of life is acquiring fame because of its medical advantages and moral contemplations.

The eating of mostly plants is one of the most important tenets of pescatarianism. This way of eating is built on grains, vegetables, fruits, and nuts. Due to their ability to lower the risk of chronic diseases like heart disease, diabetes, and cancer and their low calorie density, plant-based foods are increasingly popular. To make sure they get all the nutrients they need, pescatarians should eat a variety of fruits and vegetables.

The inclusion of fish and seafood in one's diet is another pescatarian principle. Omega-3 fatty acids, which are necessary for the health of the brain and heart, and fish and seafood are excellent sources of protein. Pescatarians are urged to pick fish and fish that are low in mercury and different poisons, as well as economically obtained. Additionally, seafood and fish consumption is regarded as more ethical than poultry and meat consumption.

The last rule of pescatarianism is the aversion of meat and poultry. Pescatarians hold the belief that eating meat and poultry is not only harmful to one's health but also unethical. Deforestation, pollution, and animal cruelty are just a few of the environmental and ethical issues that are connected to the production of meat and poultry. Pescatarians want to reduce their impact on the environment and encourage ethical food consumption by avoiding meat and poultry.

All in all, the standards of pescatarianism depend on the conviction that a plant-based diet, in blend with fish and fish, is a solid and feasible approach to everyday life. The main tenets of this diet and lifestyle are to eat mostly plant-based foods, include fish and seafood, and avoid meat and poultry. Pescatarians mean to decrease their effect on the climate, advance moral food utilization, and work on their wellbeing by following these standards

CHAPTER3

The advantages o pescatarian diet

The Advantages of increasing their intake of plant-based foods and decreasing their intake of animal products. The potential to improve overall health and lower the risk of certain chronic diseases is one of the main advantages of a piscatorial diet.

One of the essential advantages of aPescatarianism is a sort of diet that includes the utilization of fish while keeping away from meat and poultry. Following this diet is an incredible method for working on generally wellbeing and prosperity. One of the pescatarian diet is that it can assist with diminishing the gamble of coronary illness. Omega-3 fatty acids, which have been shown to improve heart health, are abundant in seafood and fish. Omega-3s can help lower blood pressure, reduce inflammation, and lower the risk of heart attack and stroke. Additionally, the majority of the significant advantages of a pescatarian diet are its excellent protein sources and low saturated fat content. Essential amino acids, which are necessary for building and maintaining muscle mass, are abundant in seafood. Additionally, fish and other seafood contain low levels of, which may further reduce the likelihood of cardiovascular disease.

A pescatarian diet's ability to assist with weight management is another advantage. Many individuals who follow a pescatarian diet find that they normally consume less calories and feel more soaked fat, making them a better option in contrast to red meat. A pescatarian diet has the added advantage of lowering the risk of heart disease. Salmon, sardines, and tuna, which contain omega-3 fatty acids, can make you feel less full after eating. This is on the grounds that plant-based food varieties and fish are for the most part less calorie-thick than meat items. Seafood's high protein content can also help you feel fuller for longer, which can help you avoid snacking between meals.

At last, a pescatarian pulse, decrease irritation, and forestall the development of blood clusters. Fish consumption twice a week has been shown to significantly lower the risk of heart disease and stroke. A pescatarian diet typically includes a lot of whole grains, fruits, and vegetables, all of which are good for the heart.

Finally, a pescatarian diet can aid in environmental preservation. Fish populations have decreased as a result of overfishing and unsustainable fishing methods, which can have a significant effect on marine ecosystems. By picking economically obtained fish and diminishing meat utilization, pescat diet can give different significant supplements that might be deficient in a common meat-weighty eating regimen. Vitamins and minerals like iron, vitamin B12, and vitamin D are abundant in seafood and fish. Whole grains, fruits, and vegetables, as well as other plant-based foods, can also supply a variety of essential nutrients for overall health and wellness. Individuals can ensure that they are consuming a diverse range of nutrients that can support optimal health by following a pescatarian diet. Pescatarians can assist in reducing their carbon footprint and promote sustainable food practices. A pescatarian diet has numerous advantages, including improved health, reduced impact on the environment, and a more sustainable food system. Pescatarianism is a kind of diet that includes devouring fish and fish while staying away from different sorts of meat like hamburger, pork, and chicken. If you're thinking about switching to a pescatarian diet, it's important to have a strategy in place to make sure you get the nutrients you need and eat a variety of delicious and filling meals.

One of the main ways to begin a pescatarian way of life is to do all necessary investigation and plan your dinners quite a bit early. This will assist you in minimizing your reliance on a single kind of fish or seafood and ensuring that you are getting all of the essential nutrients. You may likewise need to consider talking with an enrolled dietitian to assist you with making a reasonable and good feast plan.

CHAPTER4

Tips in preparing the pescatarian diet

Being open to trying new things is another important tip for starting a pescatarian lifestyle. When switching to a pescatarian diet, many people discover new recipes and cooking methods as well as new fish and seafood that they love. You might discover that you enjoy your meals more than ever before if you are willing to try new foods and experiment in the kitchen.

Last but not least, if you want to live a pescatarian lifestyle, you need to be careful about where you get your food.

Pescatarianism is a way of eating that only eats seafood and plant-based foods and doesn't eat meat from animals that live on land. Pescatarianism provides a wide range of meal planning options and is frequently adopted for ethical or health reasons. Including common pescatarian ingredients in your meals is one of the most important aspects of pescatarianism.

In a pescatarian diet, seafood is the main source of protein, and there are many different kinds of fish that are commonly eaten. Salmon, fish, and cod are famous decisions, as are shellfish like shrimp, crab, and lobster. Vegetables like asparagus, Brussels sprouts, and green beans, as well as whole grains like quinoa and brown rice, are frequently served alongside these proteins. Nuts, seeds, and legumes like chickpeas and lentils are also essential components of the pescatarian diet.

Many common pescatarian ingredients not only provide a good source of protein, but they also have a number of health benefits. Salmon, for instance, is rich in omega-3 fatty acids, which are necessary for brain and heart health. Shrimp is a decent wellspring of vitamin D, which is significant for bone and safe wellbeing, while shellfish are high in zinc, which is fundamental for wound mending and keeping a sound resistant framework. To ensure that you're getting all the essential nutrients you need to stay healthy, it's important to think about the nutritional value of the ingredients you use when planning a pescatarian meal.

In general, pescatarianism is a delicious and wholesome eating style with numerous meal options.

Normal pescatarian fixings like fish, vegetables, and entire grains are delectable, yet in addition offer an assortment of medical advantages. By integrating these fixings into your feasts, you can partake in a decent and fulfilling diet that upholds your general wellbeing and prosperity. So, if you want to try something new in the kitchen, look into pescatarian recipes and see all the delicious options that are available!

A pescatarian diet avoids all forms of meat, with the exception of fish and seafood. People who want to enjoy the benefits of a vegetarian diet while still consuming some animal protein tend to follow this diet. Pescatarian recipes are a great option for those seeking a diet that is both healthy and long-lasting because they are simple to find and prepare.

CHAPTER5

One of the most outstanding things about pescatarian recipes is that they are not difficult to make and require a couple of fixings. A straightforward salmon recipe, for instance, may only call for a few spices, lemon, and olive oil. In a similar vein, shrimp, vegetables, and a few spices can all be used to make grilled shrimp skewers. Not only are these recipes simple to prepare, but they also taste great and are healthy. Pescatarian recipes also have the advantage of being adaptable to a variety of tastes and preferences. For example, on the off chance that you could do without fish, there are numerous vegan choices that you can substitute. In a similar vein, you can spice up your recipe with chili flakes or hot sauce if you like your food spicy. Pescatarianism is a great option for people with diverse tastes and lifestyles due to its adaptability.

In conclusion, pescatarian recipes are an excellent choice for individuals who want to take pleasure in the advantages of a vegetarian diet while still consuming some animal protein. They are adaptable to various tastes and preferences, require few ingredients, and are simple to make. Pescatarianism is definitely something you should think about if you want a diet that is both healthy and long-lasting.

A diet known as pescatarianism includes seafood and fish as a source of protein while excluding meat, poultry, and other land animals. People who want to cut back on their meat consumption for health, ethical, or environmental reasons often follow this diet. While still adhering to this dietary restriction, pescatarian recipes are a great way to explore various flavor profiles and cooking techniques.

One of the most outstanding things about pescatarian recipes is that they offer a wide assortment of choices for each dinner. Try smoked salmon and avocado toast or an omelet with shrimp and vegetables for breakfast. Make a tuna or salmon salad sandwich or a bowl of seafood chowder for lunch. Even more options are available for dinner, with dishes like pan-seared scallops, baked salmon, and grilled shrimp skewers.

While some pescatarian recipes are more difficult to prepare than others, many are quick and simple to prepare. Because of this, they are ideal for quick weeknight dinners or meal preparation. Anyone can make a delicious and nutritious pescatarian dish with the right ingredients and some basic cooking skills. Whether you are a carefully prepared cook or simply beginning, there are a lot of recipes out there to suit your taste and expertise level.

A healthy and long-lasting way to eat is to follow a Pescatarian diet that is well-balanced. Fish and seafood are the primary sources of protein in a pescatarian diet, which avoids meat from land animals like beef, pork, and chicken. To keep a fair Pescatarian diet, one requirements to guarantee they are getting the right supplements to help their general wellbeing.

The abundance of omega-3 fatty acids found in a Pescatarian diet is one of its primary advantages. Fatty fish like salmon, sardines, and mackerel contain a lot of these, which are necessary for our bodies. Omega-3s are essential for supporting brain function, reducing inflammation, and maintaining a healthy heart.

However, it is essential to select mercury-free fish like sardines and wild-caught salmon.

It is essential to incorporate a variety of fruits, vegetables, and whole grains into a Pescatarian diet in order to keep it balanced. These give significant nutrients, minerals, and fiber that are fundamental for by and large wellbeing. One can include legumes, nuts, and seeds in their diet to get enough protein. In addition, it's critical to stick to whole foods for carbs and avoid highly processed foods because they can cause inflammation and long-term disease.

All in all, a fair Pescatarian diet is a solid and reasonable method for eating. It promotes a diet high in fruits, vegetables, and whole grains while also providing important nutrients like omega-3 fatty acids. Individuals can maintain a balanced Pescatarian diet that is beneficial to their overall health and well-being by adhering to these guidelines.

Consuming a variety of nutrients that are necessary for one's overall health and well-being is a necessary part of eating a balanced pescatarian diet. Omega-3 fatty acids, vitamin B12, and iron, which are typically found in fish and other seafood products, must be included in your diet as a pescatarian.

Omega-3 fatty acids are necessary for the health of the heart and brain. In order to get enough omega-3 fatty acids as a pescatarian, you need to eat fish or seafood at least twice a week. Salmon, trout, and mackerel are some of the best sources of omega-3 fatty acids. Omega-3 fatty acids can also be found in flaxseeds, walnuts, and chia seeds.

Vitamin B12 is yet another essential nutrient in a pescatarian diet. Vitamin B12 is significant for keeping up with solid nerve cells and red platelets. Pescatarians must include fish and seafood in their diets because vitamin B12 can only be found in animal products. Salmon, tuna, and shrimp are some of the best sources of vitamin B12. Beef, eggs, and dairy products are additional sources of vitamin B12.

In a balanced pescatarian diet, iron is another important nutrient. Iron is necessary for oxygen transport throughout the body and the maintenance of healthy blood cells. While iron is regularly found in red meat, it can likewise be tracked down in fish and fish items. Probably the best wellsprings of iron for pescatarians incorporate mollusks, clams, and shrimp. Lentils, spinach, and tofu are additional sources of iron. You can keep your life balanced and healthy on a pescatarian diet by including these essential nutrients.

Keeping a fair pescatarian diet is significant for the individuals who have decided to follow this dietary way of life. Pescatarianism is eating fish and seafood in addition to a vegetarian diet. This can be a sustainable and healthy way to eat, but careful planning is required to ensure that all nutrients are consumed in the right quantities. Meal planning is an important aspect of pescatarianism.

CHAPTER6

Meal planning for pescatarian diet

When planning your pescatarian meals, it's important to take into account your body's nutritional requirements. This means making sure you get enough complex carbohydrates, healthy fats, and protein. Fish and seafood are excellent sources of protein and healthy fats, but you should choose a variety of them to get a variety of nutrients. Salmon, tuna, shrimp, scallops, and mussels are excellent choices. In order to get the necessary carbohydrates, vitamins, and minerals, it's also important to include a variety of fruits, vegetables, and whole grains in your meals.

While arranging your dinners, it very well may be useful to save a period every week to plan and prepare your food ahead of time. When you're short on time, this can help you stick to your pescatarian diet and avoid unhealthy snacks and fast food. Because you can plan your meals around ingredients that can be used in multiple recipes, meal prepping can also help you save money and reduce food waste. Making a large batch of quinoa or brown rice, roasting a tray of vegetables, and grilling a variety of fish and seafood are all good meal prep options for pescatarians.

In rundown, arranging your pescatarian dinners is fundamental for keeping a reasonable and solid eating routine. By taking into account your healthful necessities and consolidating various fish and fish, natural products, vegetables, and entire grains into your dinners, you can guarantee that you are getting every one of the supplements your body needs. Dinner preparing can likewise be a useful instrument for keeping focused with your eating routine and setting aside time and cash. You can take advantage of the numerous health benefits of a pescatarian diet if you carefully plan and prepare.

It is not easy to eat a pescatarian diet that is well-balanced. When it comes to making sure you get enough nutrients, it takes careful planning and attention to detail. Here are some suggestions to help you keep a pescatarian diet healthy.

First and foremost, ensure that you consume a variety of fish. By including a variety of fish in your diet, you can ensure that you are getting a variety of nutrients because different kinds of fish provide different nutrients. Salmon, for instance, is rich in omega-3 fatty acids, while cod, a white fish, is high in protein. Choosing wild-caught fish over farmed fish can also have a big effect on how much of a nutrient you get. Wild-got fish are commonly lower in poisons and higher in supplements.

Second, nutrients derived from plants should not be overlooked. Whole grains, fruits, and vegetables are not out of the question if you follow a pescatarian diet. In point of fact, these foods may supply numerous vitamins and minerals that fish may lack. Iron is abundant in leafy greens like spinach and kale, while protein and healthy fats are abundant in nuts and seeds. By integrating an assortment of plant-based food varieties into your eating routine, you can guarantee that you are getting a balanced supplement consumption.

Last but not least, you might want to take supplements to get the nutrients you need. While it's in every case best to get your supplements from entire food sources, enhancements can be a useful device to guarantee that you are meeting your supplement needs. If you don't eat fish enough to get the recommended amount of omega-3s, for instance, omega-3 fatty acid supplements can be a good option. Be that as it may, it's vital to talk with a medical services supplier prior to beginning any new enhancement routine, as certain enhancements can collaborate with prescriptions or make unfavorable impacts.

By following these tips, you can keep a solid and adjusted pescatarian diet. Make sure to include a variety of fish and plant-based foods in your diet, and if necessary, think about taking supplements. You can make sure that your body gets all the nutrients it needs with a little planning and attention.

THE END

9 798853 105362